nour

A Step-by-Step Guide to Transforming Your Diet and Boosting Your Health.

Pete Staples

Content   Page

Step 1: Understanding Why Nourishing Your Body Matters — Introduction.

Have you ever wondered why some people seem to have boundless energy, glowing skin, and a positive outlook on life? While genetics play a role, the answer often lies in what they eat. What we put into our bodies affects not only how we look and feel, but also our risk for chronic diseases and overall longevity.

The scientific evidence linking diet and health is overwhelming and plentiful. Unhealthy diets high in processed and sugary foods have been linked to an increased risk of chronic diseases such as type 2 diabetes, heart disease, and cancer. In fact, a 2020 study published in The Lancet found that poor nutrition was responsible for 11 million deaths worldwide, making it a leading risk factor for death globally. Furthermore, a diet lacking in essential nutrients can impact cognitive function, mood regulation, and overall well-being. Clearly a poor diet can have a hug negative effect on our overall health.

On the other hand, a balanced and nutritious diet can have a positive impact on various aspects of health. A diet rich in fruits, vegetables, whole grains, and lean protein sources have been linked to a lower risk of cardiovascular disease. There is ample research that's shows that consuming foods high in vitamins and minerals can improve skin health, boost immunity, and promote healthy aging.

It's never too late to make positive changes in your diet and lifestyle to improve your overall health and well-being. In this book, we'll explore practical and evidence-based steps to help you improve your eating habits and nourish your body. By following these steps, you'll have more energy, better digestion, and a stronger immune system. Plus, you'll be reducing your risk for chronic diseases and improving your quality of life.

In the following chapters, we'll cover everything from setting your nourishment goals and intentions, to understanding the basics of nutrition, assessing your current eating habits, planning, and preparing nourishing meals and snacks, mindful eating techniques, managing cravings and emotional eating, making nourishment sustainable, and incorporating exercise and movement into your life. By the end of this book, you'll have all the tools you need to transform your diet and boost your health. Let's get started!

Key Points From Step 1: Understanding Why Nourishing Your Body Matters – Introduction.

1. Our diet has a significant impact on our overall health, including the risk for chronic diseases, cognitive function, mood regulation, and well-being.
2. Unhealthy diets high in processed and sugary foods have been linked to an increased risk of chronic diseases such as type 2 diabetes, heart disease, and cancer.
3. A balanced and nutritious diet, rich in fruits, vegetables, whole grains, and lean protein sources, has been linked to a lower risk of cardiovascular disease, improved skin health, boosted immunity, and healthy aging.
4. Poor nutrition is responsible for 11 million deaths worldwide, making it a leading risk factor for death globally.

Step 2: Setting Your Nourishment Goals and Intentions

If you want to be successful transforming your diet and boosting your health, it requires setting clear goals and intentions. Setting your nourishment goals and intentions can help you stay focused, motivated, and accountable as you make changes to your eating habits. In this chapter, we'll explore some steps to help you set your nourishment goals and intentions.

Reflect on your current state of health.

Before you start setting your nourishment goals and intentions, it's important to reflect on your current state of health. Take a moment to assess your current health status by asking yourself the following questions:

1. Are you experiencing any health issues or concerns?
2. Do you feel tired or lethargic during the day?
3. Do you struggle with your digestion?

Understanding your current health status can provide valuable insight into the types of changes you may need to make to your diet. For example, if you struggle with digestive problems, you may need to focus on incorporating more fibre-rich foods into your diet. If you struggle with tiredness and lethargic you may need to focus on your starchy carbohydrate choice and timing.

Your health is important, and once you've reflected on your health, if you're experiencing serious health issues, it's important to seek medical advice and speak to your doctor. Your doctor is there to help you, so don't hesitate to reach out to your healthcare provider if you have concerns about your health or feel you have a medical issue connected to your diet.

Identify your motivations.

Once you've reflected on your current health status, it's important to identify your motivations for nourishing your body. Think about why you want to make changes to your diet. Some common motivations include:

- ✓ Losing weight
- ✓ Gaining energy
- ✓ Improving mood
- ✓ Reducing risk of chronic disease

Understanding your motivations can help you stay committed to your goals, even when faced with challenges and setbacks.

Set specific, measurable goals.

Once you've identified your motivations, it's time to set specific, measurable goals. Setting specific goals can help you stay focused and motivated, and measuring your progress can help you stay accountable. Despite the potential benefits of setting goals, many people do not effectively utilize this practice in their personal or professional lives. But effective goal setting can help individuals clarify their priorities, stay motivated, and make progress towards their desired outcomes when done well. Here are some tips for setting specific, measurable goals:

Be realistic: Set goals that are achievable, given your current lifestyle and circumstances. Setting unrealistic goals can lead to frustration and disappointment.

Break goals into smaller steps: Breaking larger goals into smaller steps can help you stay motivated and make progress over time. For example, if your goal is to incorporate more vegetables into your diet, you could start by adding one serving of vegetables to one meal per day.

Be SMART: SMART is the acronym that stands for Specific, Measurable, Achievable, Relevant, and Time-bound. Using these criteria can help you set goals that are specific, achievable, and time bound. For example, instead of setting a goal to "eat more vegetables," you could set a SMART goal to "eat at least 3 servings of vegetables per day for the next 4 weeks."

Write down your goals.

Once you have your nourishment goals and intentions in mind, it's important to write them down. Writing down your goals can help you stay focused and committed and can serve as a reminder of what you're working towards. Here are some tips for writing down your goals:

Use positive language: Instead of focusing on what you want to avoid (e.g., "I want to stop eating junk food"), focus on what you want to achieve (e.g., "I want to eat more whole foods"). Using positive language when writing down goals can help you develop confidence, and maintain a sense of optimism and resilience as you pursue your goals.

Be specific: Use specific language to describe your goals. For example, instead of writing "eat healthier," write "eat at least 3 servings of vegetables per day." Being specific will bring you clarity to what you are trying to achieve as well as be useful when monitoring and assessing your progression. Vague goals can be hard to quantify which can give the impression of poor progression and ultimately lower your motivation. Be as specific as possible when writing your goals down and don't be afraid to modify and adapt them as you go.

Make your goals visible: Display your goals somewhere you can see them every day, such as on your refrigerator or bathroom mirror. Making your goals visible can serve as a daily reminder of what you are trying to achieve, increase your accountability, and helps you stay focused on taking the necessary steps to make progress towards your desired outcomes.

By reflecting on your current state of health, identifying your motivations, setting specific, measurable goals, and writing down your goals, you'll be well on your way to transforming your diet and boosting your health. In the next chapter, we'll explore the basics of nutrition to help you better understand how to nourish your body.

Key Points from Step 2: Setting Your Nourishment Goals and Intentions:

1. Reflect on your current state of health to identify potential health issues or concerns, such as digestive problems, and seek medical advice if necessary.
2. Identify your motivations for nourishing your body, such as losing weight, gaining energy, improving mood, or reducing the risk of chronic diseases.
3. Set specific, measurable, achievable, relevant, and time-bound (SMART) goals to stay focused, motivated, and accountable.
4. Write down your goals using positive language and specific wording, and make them visible in a place you can see every day to serve as a daily reminder and increase accountability.
5. Breaking larger goals into smaller steps can help you stay motivated and make progress over time towards your desired outcomes.

Step 3: Understanding the Basics of Nutrition

Nutrition is the foundation of a healthy body and mind. What we eat provides us with the energy and gives us the nutrients and building blocks necessary to support our bodily functions, from cellular processes to brain function. Understanding the basics of nutrition is essential for creating a healthy diet that promotes overall wellness. In this chapter, we'll explore the six essential nutrients, macronutrients, micronutrients, hydration, and how to read nutrition labels so we understand what we nutrition we are consuming.

The Six Essential Nutrients

Nutrients are substances that our bodies need to function correctly. There are six essential nutrients: carbohydrates, proteins, fats, vitamins, minerals, and water. Each nutrient plays a unique role in the body, and it's essential to consume a balanced mix of them. Each nutrient plays a unique role in the body, and it's important to consume a variety of foods that provide a mix of all six essential nutrients.

Macronutrients

Carbohydrates, proteins, and fats are referred to as macronutrients that are needed in large amounts by the body. Each macronutrient provides energy and plays a unique role in the body. It's essential to consume a balance of all three macronutrients to support overall health.

Carbohydrates provide energy for the body and are found in foods such as fruits, vegetables, grains, and dairy. Carbohydrates are broken down into glucose, which is used as the primary source of energy for the body. Complex carbohydrates, such as those found in whole grains and vegetables, provide a more sustained source of energy, while simple carbohydrates, such as those found in candy and soda, provide a quick burst of energy but can cause blood sugar spikes.

Proteins are necessary for building and repairing tissues in the body, including muscles, organs, and bones. They're made up of amino acids, which are the building blocks of protein. Complete proteins, which are found in animal products such as meat and dairy, contain all the essential amino acids that the body needs. Incomplete proteins, which are found in plant-based foods such as beans and nuts, don't contain all the essential amino acids, but can be combined with other foods to form a complete protein.

Fats are essential for the body, and they are important for several roles in the body including energy, vitamin and mineral absorption amongst numerous roles but it's important to consume them in moderation. Saturated and trans fats, which are found in foods such as red meat and fried foods, can increase the risk of heart disease, and should be limited in the diet. Unsaturated fats, which are found in foods such as nuts, seeds, and oily fish, can have a positive impact on heart health when consumed in moderation. Fats are found in foods like oils, nuts, seeds, and oily fish.

The recommended dietary guidelines suggest that carbohydrates should make up 45-65% of daily calorie intake, proteins should make up 20-35%, and fats should make up 20-35%. The amounts can depend on our age, sex, size and physical activity level.

Micronutrients

Vitamins and minerals are referred to as micronutrients because they are needed in smaller amounts in the body than macronutrients. Vitamins are organic compounds that are necessary for growth and development, while minerals are inorganic substances that are essential for bodily processes such as bone health and muscle function Foods such as fruits, vegetables, dairy, and meats are good sources of vitamins and minerals. It's important to consume a variety of foods that provide a mix of vitamins and minerals to support overall health.

Hydration

Water is essential for maintaining hydration, and it plays a crucial role in regulating bodily functions. The body needs water to transport nutrients and oxygen, remove waste, and regulate body temperature. It's essential to stay hydrated throughout the day, and the recommended amount of water varies depending on factors such as age, sex, environmental temperatures, and activity level. The general recommendation is to drink at least 2 litres of water per day, but some people may need more. Staying hydrated can also be achieved by consuming foods with high water content, such as fruits and vegetables.

Reading Nutrition Labels

Understanding how to read a nutrition label is crucial for making informed decisions about what we eat. Nutrition labels provide information about the nutrient content of foods and can help us choose foods that are nutrient-dense and support overall health. When reading a nutrition label, it's essential to look at the serving size, calories, and the amount of various nutrients, including fats, sugars, and sodium.

When reading a nutrition label, it's important not to only look at the calorie content of the food/drink and check the amount of various nutrients such as fat, sugar, and sodium. Consuming too much of these nutrients can increase the risk of chronic diseases such as heart disease and diabetes. It's also important to pay attention to serving sizes, as a single package or container may contain multiple servings.

Reading food labels is an important step in making informed decisions about the foods we consume. You can read a food label effectively by:

1. Look at the serving size to ensure that you're consuming the recommended portion.
2. Check the calories per serving and the amount of each nutrient, paying attention to the amounts of fat, sugar, and sodium. It's recommended to aim for low amounts of these nutrients to reduce the risk of chronic diseases such as heart disease and diabetes.

   When looking at food labels the following nutrients values are considered low and generally healthier:

   - Fats: 3g of fat or less per 100g/ml.
   - Sugar: 5g of total sugars or less per 100g/ml.
   - Sodium: 0.1g of sodium or less per 100g/ml (or 0.25g of salt or less per 100g/ml).

When looking at food labels the following nutrients values are considered high and generally could contribute to a unhealthier diet. Foods in have these high amounts should be used sparingly.

- High fat: A food product is considered high in fat if it contains 17.5g or more of fat per 100g.
- High sugar: A food product is considered high in sugar if it contains 22.5g or more of total sugars per 100g.
- High salt: A food product is considered high in salt if it contains 1.5g or more of salt per 100g (or 0.6g sodium).

3. Finally, take note of any added ingredients, such as preservatives or artificial colours or even nutrients you wouldn't expect in the item of food.

By taking the time to read food labels and understanding what to look for, we can make informed decisions about the foods we eat and support our overall health and wellbeing.

In this chapter, we explored the six essential nutrients, macronutrients, micronutrients, hydration, and how to read nutrition labels. Understanding the basics of nutrition is essential for creating a healthy diet that supports overall wellness. By consuming a balance of macronutrients and micronutrients and staying hydrated, we can fuel our bodies with the nutrients they need to function correctly, which ultimately results in your body and mind feeling and being healthier.

Key Points from Step 3: Understanding the Basics of Nutrition

1. There are six essential nutrients: carbohydrates, proteins, fats, vitamins, minerals, and water, and each nutrient plays a unique role in the body.
2. Carbohydrates, proteins, and fats are referred to as macronutrients that are needed in large amounts by the body. It's essential to consume a balance of all three macronutrients to support overall health.
3. Vitamins and minerals are referred to as micronutrients because they are needed in smaller amounts in the body than macronutrients.
4. Water is essential for maintaining hydration, and it plays a crucial role in regulating bodily functions. The general recommendation is to drink at least 2 litres of water per day, but some people may need more.
5. When reading a nutrition label, it's important to look at the serving size, calories, and the amount of various nutrients, including fats, sugars, and sodium, and to aim for low amounts of these nutrients to reduce the risk of chronic diseases such as heart disease and diabetes.

Step 4: Assessing Your Current Eating Habits

Eating a healthy, well-balanced diet is key to maintaining good health and preventing chronic diseases. However, many of us fall short when it comes to meeting our nutritional needs. Understanding your starting point is crucial to progressing and moving forwards. Due to the complexity people's lives, dietary choices and factors that influence them, many individuals are unaware or do not fully understand their own dietary habits, making it essential to regularly assess and record your food intake to ensure a balanced and healthy diet. In this chapter, we will explore how to assess your current eating habits, identify areas for improvement, and set goals for a healthier diet.

Keep a Food Diary

The first step in assessing your current diet is to keep a food diary. This involves recording everything you eat and drink for a few days or ideally weeks, including the time of day, portion sizes, any snacks or beverages consumed and your thoughts and mood at the time. You can use a paper journal or an app to track your intake. Personally, the clients I have worked with tend to get the best results when they write down their choices in a journal and use the a diet app to help them scan foods and meals and work out calories and nutritional content.

Keeping a food diary can help you identify patterns in your eating habits, such as whether you tend to snack at certain times of the day or consume more calories on weekends. It can also help you become more mindful of what you are eating and make more conscious choices.

Evaluate Your Intake

Once you have kept a food diary for a few days or weeks, it's time to evaluate your intake. Start by looking at the overall balance of your diet. Are you getting enough fruits and vegetables? Are you consuming too much processed or fast food? Are you consuming a mixture of protein, carbohydrate and fats? Are you consuming enough water? It's also important to look at your calorie and macronutrient intake. Are you getting the adequate amounts of protein, carbohydrates, and healthy fats? What was your overall calorie intake for the day? The recommended daily intake for each of these nutrients varies depending on factors such as age, sex, and activity level. A registered dietitian or nutritionist can help you determine your specific needs.

Identify Areas for Improvement

Based on your evaluation, identify areas for improvement. This could include increasing your intake of fruits and vegetables, reducing your consumption of processed and fast food, or making healthier snack choices.

When making changes to your diet, it's important to start small and focus on one or two areas at a time. For example, you might start by swapping out sugary beverages for water or replacing processed snacks with fresh fruit. Just look to change a couple of things that you know will have a positive influence on your diet and health.

Set Realistic Goals

Finally, set realistic goals for improving your diet. This could include aiming to consume five servings of fruits and vegetables per day, reducing your intake of added sugars, or cooking at home more often. When setting goals, it's important to make them specific, measurable, and achievable. For example, instead of setting a vague goal like "eat healthier," you might set a goal like "consume at least two servings of vegetables with every meal." Remember writing down the goals and making them visible around the house is a great way to create a daily reminder and become accountable to yourself.

Assessing your current diet is an important step in improving your health and well-being. By keeping a food diary, evaluating your intake, identifying areas for improvement, and setting realistic goals, you can make gradual changes to your diet that will have a lasting impact on your health. Remember, small changes can add up over time, so start by making one or two changes at a time and building from there.

Key Points from Step 4: Assessing Your Current Eating Habits and Identifying Areas for Improvement.

1. Keeping a food diary is a crucial step in assessing your current eating habits, as it helps identify patterns and make more conscious choices.
2. Evaluating your intake involves looking at the overall balance of your diet, including macronutrient intake, and assessing if you are consuming enough fruits, vegetables, and water.
3. Based on the evaluation, it is important to identify areas for improvement, such as increasing fruit and vegetable intake, reducing processed food consumption, or making healthier snack choices.
4. When making changes to your diet, it's important to start small and focus on one or two areas at a time.
5. Setting realistic goals that are specific, measurable, and achievable is important to ensure gradual changes and a lasting impact on your health.

Step 5: Consistency is Key! How To Nourish Your Body Daily.

Consistency is a crucial element in achieving and maintaining a healthy diet. Healthy eating is not a short-term solution but rather a long-term lifestyle change. Consistent healthy eating habits can help sustain the healthier lifestyle in the long run which will help prevent chronic diseases, maintain a healthy weight, and improve overall well-being.

There are many reasons why consistency is important in daily healthy eating goals, which include:

Habit Formation: Consistency helps to form healthy habits. When you consistently choose healthy food options, it becomes a habit, making it easier to continue the habit in the long run. It also helps to reduce cravings for unhealthy food options.

Nutritional Balance: Consistent healthy eating ensures that you receive the nutrients your body needs to function optimally. When you consistently eat nutrient-dense foods, you are providing your body with essential vitamins, minerals, and other nutrients, which can help prevent chronic diseases.

Sustainable Weight Loss: Consistency in healthy eating habits can help you achieve sustainable weight loss. Crash diets may help you lose weight quickly, but they are not sustainable, and most people regain the weight once they return to their regular eating habits. Consistent healthy eating habits can help you lose weight gradually, leading to long-term weight loss success.

Improved Digestion: Consistent healthy eating habits can help improve digestion. Eating a balanced diet with a variety of fruits, vegetables, and whole grains can help regulate bowel movements, prevent constipation, and improve overall gut health.

Increased Energy: Consistent healthy eating habits can lead to increased energy levels. When you consistently eat healthy, your body has a steady supply of nutrients to use as energy. This can help reduce fatigue and increase productivity throughout the day.

Consistency is important in daily healthy eating goals because it helps to form healthy habits, provides essential nutrients, helps to achieve sustainable weight loss, improves digestion, and increases energy levels. By making healthy eating a consistent habit, you can improve your overall well-being and health. However, being consistent with a healthy eating plan requires discipline, dedication, and planning. Here are some tips to help you stay consistent with your healthy eating plan:

Set Realistic Goals: Setting realistic goals can help you stay motivated and focused. Start by setting small, achievable goals, such as adding more vegetables to your meals or reducing your sugar intake. As you achieve these goals, you can gradually set more challenging goals.

Plan Your Meals: Planning your meals ahead of time can help you stay consistent with your healthy eating plan. Create a weekly meal plan and grocery list to ensure that you have all the ingredients you need to prepare healthy meals. Meal planning can also help you save time and money by reducing the need for takeout or fast food.

Choose Nutrient-Dense Foods: Nutrient-dense foods provide essential vitamins, minerals, and other nutrients that are important for maintaining good health. Include a variety of fruits, vegetables, whole grains, lean proteins, and healthy fats in your meals. This can help you feel satisfied and reduce cravings for unhealthy food options.

Practice Mindful Eating: Mindful eating involves paying attention to your food, your body, and your thoughts and feelings related to food. This can help you make more conscious choices about what and how much you eat. Focus on eating slowly, savoring the flavors and textures of your food, and paying attention to your hunger and fullness cues.

Avoid Skipping Meals: Skipping meals can lead to overeating and unhealthy food choices later in the day. Make sure to eat regular, balanced meals throughout the day to maintain consistent energy levels and prevent cravings.

Seek Support: Surround yourself with supportive friends and family members who share your commitment to healthy eating. Consider joining a positive community or a support group to stay motivated and accountable.

Practice Self-Compassion: Being consistent with a healthy eating plan can be challenging, and it's important to be kind and compassionate to yourself. There will be ups and downs with your progress and times you will relapse. Remember that healthy eating is a journey, not a destination, and it's okay to make mistakes along the way. Focus on progress, not perfection, learn from your mistakes, get back on track as quickly as possible and celebrate your successes.

Being consistent with a healthy eating plan requires planning, discipline, and dedication. By setting realistic goals, planning your meals, choosing nutrient-dense foods, practicing mindful eating, avoiding skipping meals, seeking support, and practicing self-compassion, you can maintain consistent healthy eating habits and improve your overall well-being.

Key Points from Step 5: Consistency is Key! How To Nourish Your Body Daily

1. Consistency is essential in achieving and maintaining a healthy diet as it helps to form healthy habits and sustain a healthier lifestyle in the long run.
2. Consistent healthy eating provides essential nutrients, helps achieve sustainable weight loss, improves digestion, and increases energy levels.
3. To stay consistent with a healthy eating plan, set realistic goals, plan your meals, choose nutrient-dense foods, practice mindful eating, avoid skipping meals, seek support, and practice self-compassion.
4. Meal planning can help save time and money by reducing the need for takeout or fast food.
5. Mindful eating can help make more conscious choices about what and how much you eat, leading to improved overall well-being.

Step 6: Planning Your Meals and Snacks for Maximum Nutrition

Knowing that eating a healthy diet is essential for maintaining good health and preventing chronic diseases is only half the battle. The other half is figuring out how to make it happen. Planning your meals and snacks can help you make healthier choices, save time, and reduce stress. In this chapter, we will explore the importance of meal planning and provide you with strategies for creating balanced meals that support your dietary goals.

The Importance of Meal Planning

Meal planning is a process of deciding in advance what you will eat and when you will eat it. It involves taking the time to plan your meals and snacks for the week ahead, including writing a grocery list and shopping for ingredients. Meal planning has several benefits, including:

Saving time: When you plan your meals in advance, you can streamline the cooking process and reduce the amount of time you spend in the kitchen. Time-saving techniques can also make healthy eating more convenient and affordable. By streamlining your meal preparation and cooking processes, you can save time and reduce stress. Here are some time-saving techniques to consider:

- ✓ Use a slow cooker or pressure cooker to cook meals while you are away.
- ✓ Pre-cook grains, such as rice or quinoa, and store in the fridge for easy use in meals.
- ✓ Consider purchasing pre-cut vegetables or salad mixes to save time during meal prep.
- ✓ Batch cook meals in advance and freeze for later use.
- ✓ Make use of leftovers by incorporating them into new meals throughout the week.

Reducing stress: By knowing what you will eat ahead of time, you can reduce the stress of deciding what to cook each day.

Saving money: When you plan your meals in advance, you can make use of ingredients you already have on hand and avoid purchasing unnecessary items.

Supporting weight management: Meal planning can help you make healthier choices and avoid overeating. Meal prepping can be a valuable tool for supporting weight management by controlling portion sizes, reducing temptation, maintaining consistency, and saving time, you can make healthy eating a habit that supports your weight loss goals.

Building a Balanced Plate

When planning your meals, one helpful tool for creating a balanced plate is the Food Plate following the 'Eat Well Guide', which has been developed in the UK by Public Health England (PHA) in collaboration with the Food Standards Agency (FSA) as a guide for healthy eating.

The Food Plate is divided into different sections: fruits, vegetables, grains, and protein.

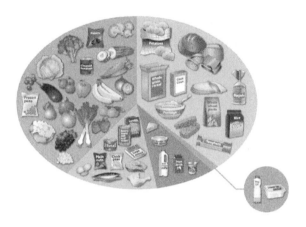

To create a balanced plate, aim fill your plate with around 35% of fruits and vegetables, around 25-35% with with whole grains, and 25-30% with lean protein and use fats and oils sparingly.

To further refine your plate, consider the following tips:

Nutrient Dense Foods:

Incorporating more nutrient-dense foods into your diet can help you meet your daily nutrient needs and get the macronutrients and micronutrients you need into your body to support your overall health and well-being. Nutrient-dense foods are foods that provide a high amount of these essential nutrients such as vitamins, minerals, fibre, protein, and healthy fats relative to their calorie content. These foods are generally considered to be healthier choices because they provide the body with the nutrients it needs to function properly without excessive calories that can contribute to weight gain or chronic diseases. Good examples include:

- ✓ **Leafy greens:** Spinach, kale, collard greens, and Swiss chard are packed with nutrients such as vitamins A, C, and K, iron, calcium, and fibre.
- ✓ **Vegetables:** Sweet potatoes, carrots, broccoli, and peppers are high in vitamins A, C, and K, fibre, and antioxidants.
- ✓ **Berries:** Blueberries, strawberries, raspberries, and blackberries are rich in antioxidants, fibre, and vitamin C.
- ✓ **Fruits:** Apples, oranges, bananas, and mangoes are high in fibre, vitamins, and minerals.
- ✓ **Nuts and seeds:** Almonds, walnuts, pumpkin seeds, and chia seeds are high in protein, healthy fats, and fibre.

- ✓ **Fish:** Salmon, tuna, and sardines are good sources of protein, omega-3 fatty acids, and vitamin D.
- ✓ **Whole grains:** Quinoa, brown rice, and oats are high in fibre, vitamins, and minerals.
- ✓ **Legumes**: Lentils, chickpeas, and black beans are high in protein, fibre, and iron.
- ✓ **Eggs:** Eggs are a good source of protein, vitamin B12, and healthy fats.
- ✓ **Dairy products:** Milk, yogurt, and cheese are high in calcium, vitamin D, and protein.

Balance macronutrients:

Look to eat a balance we have outlined with the three types of macronutrients that provide energy: carbohydrates, protein, and fat. Aim to include all three in each meal for balanced energy and satiety.

Incorporate fruits and vegetables:

Fruits and vegetables are packed with vitamins, minerals, and fibre. Aim for at least five servings per day.

Choose healthy fats: Healthy fats, such as those found in nuts, seeds, avocados, and fatty fish, can help reduce inflammation and support heart health.

Meal Planning Strategies

Meal prep strategies involve preparing and cooking meals in advance, usually in larger quantities, for consumption throughout the week. This can involve planning menus, buying groceries, cooking, and portioning meals into containers. Meal prep strategies are becoming increasingly popular as they offer a range of benefits. Meal prep can save time and money by reducing the need for frequent trips to the grocery store and takeout meals. When meal prepping it can help people to eat healthier by providing balanced and nutritious meals that are easy to grab and go. Finally, meal prep can reduce stress and anxiety associated with meal planning and cooking, making it easier to stick to healthy eating habits.

There are several strategies you can use to make meal planning easier:

1. **Weekly meal planning:** Set aside time each week to plan your meals for the week ahead. Write down your menu and create a grocery list.

2. **Batch cooking:** Cook large batches of food and portion them out for the week ahead. This can be helpful for busy weeks when you don't have much time to cook.

3. **Meal prep for the week:** Spend time on the weekends prepping ingredients for the week ahead. This might include washing and chopping vegetables or cooking grains and proteins.

4. **Freezing meals:** Cook extra portions of meals and freeze them for later use. This can be helpful for nights when you don't feel like cooking.

While setting up a meal prep routine may take some initial time and effort, it ultimately saves time and offers numerous benefits in the long run and is well worth the energy to do it.

Planning Snacks for Maximum Nutrition

Snacks can be an important part of your diet, providing energy and nutrients throughout the day. However, it's essential to choose healthy snacks that support your dietary goals. Here are some tips for planning snacks for maximum nutrition:

Healthy Snack Options: Choose snacks that are high in protein, fibre, and healthy fats. Here are some examples:

- ✓ A handful of nuts or seeds
- ✓ A piece of fruit with nut butter
- ✓ Greek yogurt with berries and granola
- ✓ Hummus with veggies or whole-grain crackers
- ✓ Hard-boiled eggs
- ✓ Cottage cheese with fruit
- ✓ Roasted chickpeas or edamame

How to Choose Snacks That Support Your Dietary Goals: When choosing snacks, consider your dietary goals. If you're trying to lose weight, aim for snacks that are low in calories and high in protein and fibre. If you're trying to build muscle or gain weight, choose snacks that are higher in calories and protein.

Portion Control for Snacks: While snacks can be a healthy part of your diet, it's essential to practice portion control. Snacks should be small and satisfying, not a full meal. Here are some tips for practicing portion control:

1. Use measuring cups or a food scale to measure out portions.
2. Avoid eating straight out of the package. Instead, portion out your snack onto a plate or bowl.
3. Consider pre-portioned snacks, such as snack packs or single-serving containers.

By planning healthy snacks that support your dietary goals and practicing portion control, you can ensure that snacks are a nutritious and satisfying part of your diet.

Making Healthy Choices While Eating Out

Eating out can be a challenge when trying to maintain a healthy diet, but it's not impossible. With a little planning and mindfulness, you can make healthy choices while enjoying meals out.

Strategies for Choosing Healthy Options While Eating Out:

- ✓ Look for menu items that are grilled, baked, or steamed instead of fried or sautéed.
- ✓ Choose dishes that are rich in vegetables, lean protein, and whole grains.
- ✓ Ask for dressings, sauces, and condiments on the side to control portions and reduce calories.
- ✓ Choose water or unsweetened beverages instead of sugary drinks or alcohol.
- ✓ Be mindful of portion sizes and consider splitting a meal or taking leftovers home.

Tips for Navigating Menus and Portion Sizes:

- ✓ Do your research and look at the menu ahead of time. Most, if not all restaurants have their menus available online to view.

- ✓ Ask your server about ingredients or cooking methods, and request modifications or substitutions as needed.
- ✓ Be aware that restaurant portions are often larger than necessary. Consider sharing a dish or ordering an appetizer as a meal.
- ✓ Avoid buffets or all-you-can-eat restaurants, as it can be challenging to control portions.

Managing Special Dietary Needs While Eating Out

If you have special dietary needs, such as food allergies or intolerances, it's important to communicate with your server and ask questions about ingredients and preparation methods. Here are some tips for managing special dietary needs while eating out:

- ✓ Research menus online before visiting the restaurant to find options that meet your needs.
- ✓ Call ahead to ask about menu items and preparation methods.
- ✓ Be prepared to ask questions and communicate your needs to your server.

✓ Consider bringing your own snacks or condiments if needed.

By following these strategies and tips, you can make healthy choices while eating out without sacrificing taste or enjoyment. Remember that it's okay to indulge occasionally, but making mindful choices most of the time can help you maintain a healthy and balanced diet.

Creating a Grocery List

Creating a grocery list is an essential step in planning your meals and ensuring that you have the ingredients you need to make healthy choices. There are numerous benefits of creating a grocery list and tips for making one:

Benefits of Creating a Grocery List:

✓ Saves time and reduces stress by helping you plan meals and avoid multiple trips to the store.
✓ Helps you stick to your budget and avoid impulse purchases.
✓ Ensures that you have the ingredients you need to make healthy meals and snacks.

✓ Reduces food waste by allowing you to plan meals based on what you already have in your pantry or fridge.

How to Successfully Make a Grocery List:

✓ Start by planning your meals for the week. Consider the recipes you want to make and the ingredients you will need.

✓ Check your pantry, fridge, and freezer to see what ingredients you already have on hand.

✓ Make a list of the ingredients you need to buy, organized by category (e.g., produce, dairy, meats, etc.).

✓ Consider adding healthy snacks, such as fruits and nuts, to your list.

✓ Use a mobile app or a pen and paper to create your list.

Tips for Sticking to Your List and Avoiding Impulse Purchases:

✓ Stick to your list and avoid buying items that are not on it.

- ✓ Shop the perimeter of the store, where the fresh produce, meats, and dairy products are located.
- ✓ Avoid the middle aisles, where processed and packaged foods are often located.
- ✓ Don't shop when you're hungry, as this can lead to impulse purchases.
- ✓ Consider buying generic or store-brand items instead of brand-name products to save money.

By creating a grocery list, you can plan your meals, save time and money, and make healthy choices at the grocery store. Don't forget to check your list before you leave for the store and stick to it while you shop.

Throughout this chapter we have looked at why and how meal prepping and planning as well as the factors around it is important and the essential steps you need to take to help you in transforming your diet and boosting your health. By taking the time to plan your meals, you can ensure that you're eating a variety of nutrient-dense foods, balancing macronutrients, and incorporating fruits and vegetables. Planning your snacks and making healthy choices while eating out can also help you stay on track with your dietary goals.

Key Points from Step 6: Planning Your Meals and Snacks for Maximum Nutrition

1. Meal planning is important for saving time, reducing stress, saving money, and supporting weight management.
2. To create a balanced plate, aim for 35% fruits and vegetables, 25-35% whole grains, and 25-30% lean protein, with fats and oils used sparingly.
3. Nutrient-dense foods, such as leafy greens, vegetables, berries, nuts and seeds, fish, whole grains, eggs, and dairy products, can help meet daily nutrient needs and support overall health and well-being.
4. Balancing macronutrients, incorporating fruits and vegetables, and choosing healthy fats are helpful strategies for building a balanced plate.
5. Meal planning strategies, such as meal prepping, can save time and money, and can help ensure that healthy meals are available throughout the week.

Step 7: Cooking and Preparing Nourishing Meals and Snacks

We know eating a balanced and nutritious diet is one of the most important things you can do for your health. But it's not always easy to know what to eat, how to prepare it, and how to make healthy choices that fit your lifestyle. That's where cooking and preparing meals and snacks come in. By taking control of what you eat and how you prepare it, you can transform your diet and boost your health.

The Importance of Cooking and Preparing Meals and Snacks:

Cooking and preparing food at home also promotes healthy eating habits, reduces the intake of processed foods, and can save money in the long run. Furthermore, cooking and preparing food can be a rewarding and enjoyable experience, providing a sense of accomplishment and satisfaction in creating something from scratch. In this context, it is important to understand the benefits of cooking and preparing meals and snacks and how they can positively impact our health and well-being. Cooking and preparing meals and snacks have numerous benefits, including:

- ✓ Control over the ingredients: When you cook and prepare your meals and snacks, you know exactly what goes into them. You can avoid processed foods, unhealthy fats, and excessive amounts of sugar and salt.
- ✓ Cost-effective: Cooking at home is generally more cost-effective than eating out, especially if you buy ingredients in bulk or on sale.
- ✓ Portion control: Cooking and preparing your meals and snacks can help you control portion sizes and reduce food waste.
- ✓ Time-saving: While cooking and preparing meals and snacks may take some time upfront, it can save you time in the long run. Batch cooking and meal prep can help you have healthy meals and snacks ready to go when you need them.

How Cooking and Preparing Meals and Snacks Can Help with Weight Management

Cooking and preparing your meals and snacks can also help with weight management and there is ample research and to support this. By controlling the ingredients and portion sizes, you can reduce the number of calories you consume. Additionally, cooking at home often leads to eating fewer calories than eating out at restaurants, which tend to serve larger portions and higher calorie dishes.

Navigating the Kitchen and Filling the Kitchen Cupboards:

Having the right tools and appliances in your kitchen can make cooking and preparing meals and snacks easier and more enjoyable. It can save time and effort when you have the appropriate kitchen tools and appliances for the meal you are trying to prepare and cook. Some essential tools and appliances include:

- ✓ Cutting board and knives
- ✓ Mixing bowls
- ✓ Measuring cups and spoons
- ✓ Pots and pans
- ✓ Blender or food processor
- ✓ Oven, Slow Cooker, Air Fryer

Stocking your kitchen cupboards with healthy ingredients can make cooking and preparing meals and snacks easier and more convenient. Some essentials to have on hand include:

- ✓ Whole grains: brown rice, quinoa, oats, and whole-wheat pasta
- ✓ Canned or dried beans: black beans, chickpeas, and lentils

- ✓ Nuts and seeds: almonds, walnuts, chia seeds, and flaxseeds
- ✓ Healthy fats: olive oil, coconut oil, and avocado
- ✓ Herbs and spices: garlic, ginger, turmeric, cumin, and paprika

Understanding Cooking Techniques and Methods

Understanding basic cooking techniques and methods can help you cook and prepare healthy meals and snacks. Some techniques to know include:

- ✓ Baking: cooking food in an oven, often with a coating of breadcrumbs or batter
- ✓ Roasting: cooking food in an oven, often with oil or seasoning
- ✓ Sautéing: cooking food quickly in a pan with a small amount of oil or butter
- ✓ Grilling: cooking food over an open flame, often with a marinade or seasoning
- ✓ Steaming: cooking food over boiling water, often in a basket or steamer

Prepping Healthy Meals:

Preparing healthy meals can seem daunting, especially if you're new to meal prep. However, with the right approach, it can become a seamless part of your routine. Here are some tips to help you prep healthy meals with ease:

✓ **Start small:** If you're new to meal prep, start by prepping just one meal or snack per day. Once you get the hang of it, you can gradually increase the number of meals you prep each week.

✓ **Choose recipes wisely:** Look for recipes that are easy to prepare and can be made in large batches. One-pot meals and sheet pan dinners are great options for easy and efficient meal prep.

✓ Invest in quality storage containers: Choose containers that are microwave-safe, leak-proof, and stackable. Glass containers are a great choice, as they are durable and don't absorb odours or stains.

- ✓ **Keep it simple**: Don't overcomplicate your meals with too many ingredients or complex recipes. Stick to simple, wholesome ingredients and flavours that you enjoy.
- ✓ **Prep ingredients in advance:** Spend some time on the weekend or your day off chopping vegetables, cooking grains, and prepping proteins. This can help streamline the cooking process during the week.
- ✓ **Use tools and appliances:** Kitchen tools such as food processors, blenders, and slow cookers can be great time-savers. Consider investing in these tools to make meal prep easier.
- ✓ **Store food properly:** Proper storage is key to keeping your prepped meals fresh and safe to eat. Store foods in airtight containers in the refrigerator or freezer, and label them with the date.

By following these tips, you can simplify the meal prep process and make it a seamless part of your healthy lifestyle.

Cooking and Preparing Techniques:

Cooking and preparing techniques play a crucial role in determining the nutritional value and taste of your meals. The way in which food is cooked can significantly affect the nutrient content and digestibility of the food. For instance, overcooking vegetables can lead to a loss of nutrients, while undercooking meats can increase the risk of foodborne illness. On the other hand, cooking methods such as steaming, baking, and grilling can help to retain nutrients and flavours in food. By choosing healthy cooking and preparing techniques and incorporating flavourful ingredients, people can improve the overall quality and nutritional value of their meals, making healthy eating a more enjoyable experience. Here are some techniques to help you cook and prepare healthy, nourishing meals and snacks:

Roasting: Roasting is a great way to bring out the natural flavours of vegetables and fruits. It's also a simple and healthy cooking method that requires little added fat. To roast vegetables, simply toss them with a little bit of olive oil and your favourite seasonings, and roast in the oven until they are tender and golden brown.

Steaming: Steaming is a gentle cooking method that helps to retain the natural flavour and nutrients of foods. It's also a great way to cook vegetables without added fat. To steam vegetables, simply place them in a steamer basket over a pot of boiling water and cook until they are tender.

Grilling: Grilling is a great way to add flavor to meats and vegetables without adding extra fat. It's also a quick and easy cooking method that's perfect for busy weeknights. To grill vegetables, brush them with a little bit of olive oil and your favorite seasonings, and grill until they are tender and lightly charred.

Stir-frying: Stir-frying is a quick and easy cooking method that's perfect for busy weeknights. It's also a great way to cook vegetables and meats quickly without adding extra fat. To stir-fry, simply heat a little bit of oil in a wok or skillet, add your ingredients, and cook until they are tender.

Baking: Baking is a healthy cooking method that requires little added fat. It's also a great way to cook proteins such as fish, chicken, and tofu. To bake, simply season your protein with your favourite seasonings, and bake in the oven until it is cooked through.

If you are not be very experienced cooking, some of these methods and cooking in general can feel daunting. But learning to cook is an important life skill and with a little bit of practice and persistence and incorporating these cooking and preparing techniques into your meal prep routine, you can create healthy and delicious meals and snacks that support your dietary goals which will give you a sense of accomplishment and control.

Quick and Easy Meals and Snacks:

When it comes to healthy eating, convenience can be key. Quick and easy meals and snacks can be a lifesaver when you're short on time or just don't feel like cooking. Here are some tips for creating quick and easy meals and snacks that are also nourishing and delicious:

Remember Meal Prep: One of the best ways to ensure you have healthy meals and snacks on hand is to meal prep. Meal prepping comes into its own and reaps the benefits after a long day, that you normally would have the feeling like you don't want to cook because you're tired, only to remember you don't have to worry because its already been prepped and sorted. Spend a few hours each week prepping ingredients, cooking proteins, and portioning out meals and snacks. This way, you can easily grab a pre-made meal or snack when you're in a rush.

Smoothies: Smoothies are a quick and easy way to get a variety of nutrients in one meal or snack. Simply blend together your favourite fruits, vegetables, protein powder, and liquid, and you've got a nutritious meal or snack in minutes. The trick is not to just pack your smoothie with just fruit and just consume a sugary drink. Think about different ingredients you could add to your smoothie which will offer different nutrients. Why not try this one:

Green Protein Smoothie:
- 1 cup of fresh spinach
- 1 medium banana
- 1/2 avocado
- 1 scoop of vanilla protein powder
- 1/2 cup of unsweetened almond milk
- 1/2 cup of ice
- 1 teaspoon of chia seeds

Overnight Oats: Overnight oats are a great option for a quick and easy breakfast or snack. Simply mix oats, milk or yogurt, and your favourite toppings, and let it sit in the fridge overnight. In the morning, you'll have a delicious and filling breakfast or snack ready to go.

Buddha Bowls: Buddha bowls are a popular trend in healthy eating, and for good reason. They're quick and easy to make and can be customized with a variety of ingredients to suit your taste. Simply layer together cooked grains, proteins, vegetables, and a healthy dressing, and you've got a delicious and nourishing meal in minutes.

Snack Plates: Snack plates are a fun and easy way to get a variety of nutrients in one snack. Simply assemble a plate with a variety of healthy snacks, such as fruit, vegetables, nuts, and hummus. This way, you can satisfy your hunger quickly and easily without resorting to unhealthy options.

By incorporating these quick and easy meals and snacks into your routine, you can stay on track with your dietary goals even when you're short on time. Remember, healthy eating doesn't have to be time-consuming or complicated. With a little bit of planning and creativity, you can create nourishing and delicious meals and snacks that fit into your busy lifestyle.

Cooking for Special Dietary Needs:

Cooking for special dietary needs can seem daunting and can add a layer of complexity to your diet and choices, but with a little bit of planning and creativity, it's possible to create nourishing and delicious meals that cater to a variety of dietary restrictions. Here are some tips for cooking for special dietary needs:

Know the Dietary Restrictions: Before you start cooking, make sure you understand the dietary restrictions of the person or people you are cooking for. This may include allergies, intolerances, or lifestyle choices such as vegetarianism or veganism. Do a little research around the dietary restrictions to help you make the best choices and understand the different foods and recipes you can try.

Adapt Recipes: Once you know the dietary restrictions, adapt recipes to suit those needs. This may mean substituting ingredients, such as using gluten-free flour instead of wheat flour, or omitting certain ingredients altogether.

Experiment with New Ingredients: Cooking for special dietary needs can be an opportunity to try out new ingredients and cooking techniques. For example, if you're cooking for someone who is lactose intolerant, you may want to experiment with non-dairy milk alternatives such as almond milk or soy milk.

Keep it Simple: Don't feel like you need to make complicated dishes to accommodate special dietary needs. Simple meals such as grilled chicken with roasted vegetables or stir-fried tofu and veggies can be both delicious and satisfying.

Get Creative with Flavours: Special dietary needs can be an opportunity to experiment with new flavours and seasonings. Try using herbs and spices to add flavour to dishes, or experiment with new sauces and dressings.

Seek Inspiration: There are many resources available for cooking for special dietary needs, including cookbooks, online recipes, and food blogs. Don't be afraid to seek inspiration from these sources and adapt recipes to suit your needs.

Cooking for special dietary needs requires a bit of extra effort and attention, but it can also be a rewarding and creative process. By understanding the dietary restrictions of those you are cooking for, adapting recipes to suit their needs, experimenting with new ingredients and flavours, and seeking inspiration from a variety of sources, you can create delicious and nourishing meals that cater to a variety of dietary needs. Whether you are cooking for yourself or for others, remember that with a little bit of planning and creativity, you can enjoy healthy and satisfying meals that are both delicious and accommodating.

In this chapter, we covered the importance of cooking and preparing nourishing meals and snacks. We discussed various cooking and preparation techniques, quick and easy meal and snack ideas, and tips for cooking for special dietary needs. By cooking and preparing your own meals and snacks, you have the power to control the ingredients and ensure that you are consuming the nutrients your body needs to thrive. Planning and preparing meals and snacks in advance can save time and money and make healthy eating a more manageable part of your daily routine.

Remember to focus on nutrient-dense ingredients, experiment with new flavours and cooking techniques, and take the time to enjoy the process of preparing nourishing meals and snacks. By making cooking and preparing meals and snacks a priority, you can take charge of your health and wellbeing and create a positive relationship with food.

Key Points from Step 7: Cooking and Preparing Nourishing Meals and Snacks

1. Cooking and preparing meals and snacks at home promotes healthy eating habits, reduces the intake of processed foods, and can save money in the long run.
2. Cooking and preparing meals and snacks provide control over the ingredients, which helps avoid unhealthy fats, sugar, and salt.
3. Cooking and preparing meals and snacks help with weight management by reducing the number of calories consumed and eating fewer calories than eating out.
4. Having essential kitchen tools and appliances and healthy ingredients stocked in the kitchen cupboards makes cooking and preparing meals and snacks easier and more convenient.
5. Understanding basic cooking techniques and methods and meal prep tips can help prep healthy meals easily, with proper storage for maintaining freshness and safety.

Step 8: Mindful Eating: Techniques for Staying Present and Focused During Meals

Eating is something we do multiple times a day, but we often do it without much thought or attention. Mindful eating is a practice that encourages us to be more present and focused during meals, helping us to connect with our food, our bodies, and our senses. In today's world there is a high likelihood that you spend little to no time eating at a table with family. Instead, we are distracted by screens, emails, and messages whilst we eat, and it can have negative consequences. By eating mindfully, we can transform our relationship with food and boost our overall health and well-being as well as build a more positive relationship with our family and friends.

Understanding Mindful Eating:

Mindful eating is the practice of bringing awareness and attention to the act of eating. It involves paying attention to the physical sensations of hunger and fullness, as well as the taste, texture, and smell of the food. Mindful eating can help us to appreciate and enjoy our food more, while also preventing overeating and improving digestion. Some benefits of mindful eating include:

- ✓ Reducing stress and anxiety related to food and eating.
- ✓ Enhancing the pleasure and satisfaction of eating
- ✓ Improving digestion and nutrient absorption
- ✓ Preventing overeating and weight gain
- ✓ Boosting overall health and well-being

Techniques for Practicing Mindful Eating:

There are several techniques that can help us to practice mindful eating. These include:

1. **Paying attention to hunger and fullness cues:** Before eating, take a moment to check in with your body and assess how hungry you are. During the meal, pay attention to how full you are feeling and stop eating when you are satisfied.

2. **Eating slowly and savouring each bite:** Take your time with each bite, chewing slowly and savouring the taste and texture of the food. This can help you to feel more satisfied and prevent overeating.

3. **Avoiding distractions while eating:** Avoid watching TV, scrolling through your phone, or engaging in other activities while eating. Instead, focus on the act of eating and being present with your food. Try turning off your phone or putting into another room. Make sure the dining room table is clear and set to be eaten at.

4. **Engaging all senses while eating:** Pay attention to the look of, the smells, sounds and textures of the food. This can help you to fully engage with the experience of eating and enhance your enjoyment of the food. It is also a useful tactic to use to help you to eat slowly.

5. **Practicing gratitude for food:** Take a moment before eating to express gratitude for the food you are about to eat. This can help you to cultivate a deeper appreciation for the food and the nourishment it provides.

Tips for Incorporating Mindful Eating into Your Daily Routine:

Incorporating mindful eating into your daily routine can take practice and patience, but the effort can help you develop a healthier and more balanced relationship with food, allowing you to better appreciate the food you eat, make more conscious choices about what you consume, and ultimately feel more satisfied with your meals. Here are some tips to help you practice mindful eating daily:

Plan ahead for meals and snacks: Having healthy and nourishing food readily available can help you to make mindful eating choices.

Create an appropriate eating environment: Choose a quiet and comfortable space to eat, free from distractions or interruptions. Set the dining room table.

Start small and gradually build up to mindful eating: Begin by incorporating one or two mindful eating techniques into your meals, and gradually add more as you become more comfortable.

Be patient with yourself and avoid self-judgment: Mindful eating is a practice, and it takes time and effort to develop. Be kind and patient with yourself as you learn and grow.

Common Obstacles to Mindful Eating:

Despite the benefits of mindful eating, there are several common obstacles that can make it challenging to incorporate into your daily routine. Here are some of the most common obstacles and importantly some ideas and strategies for overcoming them:

Time constraints and busy schedules: One of the biggest obstacles to mindful eating is finding the time to prepare and enjoy meals. Many of us have busy schedules that leave little time for meal planning and preparation. As a result, we may resort to fast food or convenience meals, which can be high in calories, unhealthy, and unsatisfying.

To overcome this obstacle, it's important to prioritize mealtime and make it a priority. Set aside time each week to plan your meals and snacks and consider meal prepping to save time during the week. Try to create a peaceful environment for eating, free from distractions, so you can fully focus on the act of eating.

Emotional Eating:. Many of us turn to food for comfort or to cope with stress, anxiety, or other emotions. This can lead to mindless eating, where we eat without paying attention to our hunger or fullness cues.

To overcome emotional eating, it's important to practice self-care and find alternative ways to cope with emotions. This could include practicing mindfulness or meditation, getting regular exercise, or seeking support from friends, family, or a therapist.

Social pressure to overeat: Social events and gatherings can make it difficult to practice mindful eating. We may feel pressure to eat more than we need to or indulge in unhealthy foods to fit in with the group.

To overcome social pressure to overeat, it's important to be mindful of your own needs and boundaries. Set realistic goals for yourself, such as only indulging in one small treat or opting for a healthier option on the menu. Practice saying no when you feel uncomfortable or pressured to overeat and focus on enjoying the company and conversation instead of the food.

Lack of awareness of hunger and fullness cues: Many of us have lost touch with our body's natural hunger and fullness cues, which can make it difficult to practice mindful eating.

To overcome this obstacle, it's important to tune in to your body and pay attention to how you feel before, during, and after meals. Take a moment to assess your hunger and fullness before eating and pause during the meal to check in with your body and see if you are still hungry or full. Over time, this can help you to better understand your body's needs and develop a more intuitive approach to eating.

Mindful Eating

Mindful eating is a powerful tool for transforming your relationship with food and improving your overall health and well-being. While there are common obstacles to practicing mindful eating, with patience, practice, and persistence, it is possible to overcome these challenges and reap the benefits of mindful eating. By prioritizing mealtime, practicing self-care, setting realistic goals, and tuning in to your body's needs, you can cultivate a more mindful approach to eating and enjoy the many benefits that come with it. While it can be challenging to incorporate mindful eating into your daily routine, the benefits are well worth the effort. By overcoming common obstacles such as time constraints, emotional eating, social pressure, and lack of awareness of hunger and fullness cues, you can develop a more mindful approach to eating and enjoy the many benefits that come with it.

Remember, mindful eating is not a diet or a quick fix solution. It is a lifelong practice that requires patience, persistence, and self-compassion. By approaching mindful eating with an open mind and a willingness to learn and grow, you can transform your relationship with food and enjoy a healthier life.

Key Points from Step 8: Mindful Eating: Techniques for Staying Present and Focused During Meals

1. Mindful eating involves paying attention to physical sensations of hunger and fullness, taste, texture, and smell of food. It can help to appreciate food more, prevent overeating, and improve digestion and nutrient absorption.
2. Techniques for practicing mindful eating include paying attention to hunger and fullness cues, eating slowly, avoiding distractions, engaging all senses while eating, and practicing gratitude for food.
3. Tips for incorporating mindful eating into daily routine include planning ahead for meals and snacks, creating an appropriate eating environment, starting small, and being patient with oneself.
4. Common obstacles to mindful eating are time constraints, emotional eating, and social pressure to overeat. Strategies for overcoming these obstacles include prioritizing mealtime, practicing self-care, setting realistic goals, saying no, and focusing on enjoying the company and conversation.
5. Eating mindfully can transform our relationship with food, boost overall health and well-being, and build a more positive relationship with family and friends.

Step 9: Mental Health and Food: Nourishing Your Body to Support Mental Health

In today's fast-paced world, mental health issues like anxiety and depression are becoming increasingly common. While there are many factors that can contribute to mental health issues, one factor that is often overlooked is the role of nutrition. The food we eat plays a crucial role in our overall health, and it turns out that it can also have a significant impact on our mental health. In this chapter, we'll explore the connection between mental health and nutrition and discuss how making changes to our diet can improve our mood, energy levels, and overall well-being.

The Role of Nutrients in Brain Function

Certain nutrients are crucial for brain health, and deficiencies in these nutrients can lead to mental health issues like depression and anxiety. Carbohydrate rich foods such as whole gain foods as well as omega-3 fatty acids, found in fatty fish like salmon and sardines, are important for brain function and have been shown to improve symptoms of depression. B vitamins, found in foods like leafy greens and legumes, are also important for brain health and can help improve cognitive function. Antioxidants, found in colourful fruits and vegetables, protect the brain from oxidative stress and inflammation. A lack of these nutrients can result in poor mood, lack of concentration, irritability, and brain fog, which demonstrates the importance of a nutrient dense, varied, and balanced approach to your diet.

The Impact of Sugar and Processed Foods on Mood and Energy

In addition to getting enough of the right nutrients, it's also important to avoid foods that can have a negative impact on mental health. High-sugar diets have been linked to mood swings and can lead to a crash in energy levels. Processed foods, which are often high in sugar and unhealthy fats, can also lead to brain fog and decreased cognitive function. By focusing on whole foods and avoiding processed foods and added sugars, you can improve your mood and energy levels.

Gut Health and Mental Health

The gut-brain connection is becoming increasingly well-understood, and it turns out that the health of our gut can have a significant impact on our mental health. The trillions of bacteria in our gut, collectively known as the gut microbiome, play a crucial role in regulating mood and anxiety. By eating a diet rich in fibre and fermented foods, like sauerkraut and kimchi, you can support a healthy gut microbiome and improve your mental health.

Mindful Eating for Improved Mental Health

Finally, practicing mindful eating can be a powerful tool for improving mental health. By eating slowly and mindfully, you can improve your awareness of hunger and fullness cues and reduce stress around food. Mindful eating can also help you savour your food more and improve your overall relationship with food. Techniques like breathing exercises and gratitude practices can help you stay present and focused during meals and improve your mental well-being.

By nourishing your body with nutrient-dense foods and avoiding processed foods and added sugars, you can support your mental health and improve your mood and energy levels. Additionally, by supporting a healthy gut microbiome and practicing mindful eating, you can further improve your mental well-being. By making small changes to your diet and lifestyle, you can take control of your mental health and feel your best.

Key Points from Step 9: Mental Health and Food: Nourishing Your Body to Support Mental Health

1. Certain nutrients, such as omega-3 fatty acids, B vitamins, and antioxidants, are crucial for brain health and deficiencies in these nutrients can lead to mental health issues like depression and anxiety.
2. High-sugar diets and processed foods can have a negative impact on mental health, leading to mood swings, decreased cognitive function, and a crash in energy levels.
3. The gut-brain connection is increasingly understood, and a healthy gut microbiome is crucial for regulating mood and anxiety. Eating a diet rich in fibre and fermented foods can support a healthy gut microbiome.
4. Mindful eating can be a powerful tool for improving mental health by improving awareness of hunger and fullness cues, reducing stress around food, and improving the overall relationship with food.
5. By making small changes to your diet and lifestyle, such as eating nutrient-dense foods, avoiding processed foods and added sugars, supporting a healthy gut microbiome, and practicing mindful eating, you can take control of your mental health and improve your mood and energy levels.

Step 10: Managing Cravings and Emotional Eating

Cravings and emotional eating are common struggles that many people face in their journey to improve their diet and health. Cravings are the intense desire to consume a specific type of food, while emotional eating is the act of eating in response to emotions, rather than hunger. These behaviours can have a negative impact on health, leading to weight gain, poor nutrition, and increased risk of chronic diseases we are trying to avoid. In this chapter, we will explore strategies for managing cravings and emotional eating, so that you can stay on track with your health goals.

Understanding Cravings

Cravings are a natural part of the human experience, but understanding what causes them can help you manage them better. Cravings can be caused by a variety of factors, including hormonal changes, nutrient deficiencies, stress, and environmental cues. Different types of cravings include physical cravings, such as those for sugar or caffeine, and psychological cravings, such as those for comfort foods. Cravings can also be triggered by certain situations, such as social events or boredom.

Cravings can have a negative impact on health, as they often lead to overconsumption of unhealthy foods. This can result in weight gain, poor nutrition, and increased risk of chronic diseases and certain cancers. Understanding your triggers for cravings can help you identify when they are likely to occur and take steps to manage them.

Understanding Emotional Eating

Emotional eating is the act of eating in response to emotions, rather than hunger. Emotional eating can be triggered by a variety of emotions, including stress, anxiety, boredom, and sadness. Emotional eating can lead to overeating, as individuals may consume large amounts of food in an attempt to soothe their emotions. This can lead to weight gain and poor nutrition, as individuals may consume high-calorie, low-nutrient foods when emotional.

It is important to identify your triggers for emotional eating, as this can help you take steps to manage this behaviour.

Strategies for Managing Cravings and Emotional Eating

There are several strategies you can use to manage cravings and emotional eating:

Mindful Eating: As we covered in the previous chapter, Mindful eating is the practice of paying attention to your food and eating habits. Practicing being present and fully engaged in the act of eating, rather than eating mindlessly. Mindful eating can help you identify when you are hungry and when you are full, which can prevent overeating. It can also help you identify your triggers for cravings and emotional eating.

The next time you go to practice mindful eating, start by taking a few deep breaths before you eat. Then, take a moment to observe your food and appreciate its colours, textures, and smells. Take small bites and chew slowly, Try to savour the flavours and textures of your food. Pay attention to how your body feels as you eat and stop eating when you feel satisfied.

Healthy Alternatives: One way to manage cravings is to find healthy alternatives to the foods you crave. For example, if you are craving something sweet, try eating a piece of fruit or a small serving of dark chocolate. If you are craving something crunchy, try snacking on raw vegetables or whole-grain crackers.

Incorporating healthy alternatives into your diet can help you manage cravings and improve your overall nutrition. When choosing healthy alternatives, look for foods that are high in nutrients and low in calories, such as fruits, vegetables, whole grains, and lean protein sources. Remember try to pick from nutrient dense foods.

Addressing Emotional Eating: To manage emotional eating, it is important to find alternative ways to cope with your emotions. This may include practicing relaxation techniques such as deep breathing or meditation, engaging in physical activity such as walking or working out, or reaching out to a support system such as friends, family, or a therapist. When you feel the urge to eat in response to emotions, try to pause and identify what you are feeling. Then, choose an alternative coping mechanism that will help you manage your emotions without turning to food.

Planning Ahead: As you've probably noticed by now, planning is an effective strategy for most things we are trying to achieve and managing cravings and emotional eating is no different. This may involve creating a meal plan for the week, stocking your kitchen with healthy snacks, or having a plan in place for how to handle social events or other situations that may trigger cravings or emotional eating. When you have a plan in place, you are more likely to stick to your goals and avoid unhealthy behaviours.

Practicing Self-Compassion: Remember that these behaviours are normal and natural, and that it is okay to have slip-ups or setbacks. Instead of beating yourself up for giving in to a craving or emotional eating, try to approach these situations with kindness and understanding. Focus on the progress you have made towards managing these behaviours and use setbacks as an opportunity to learn and grow.

Managing cravings and emotional eating is an important step towards improving your diet and overall health. By understanding what causes these behaviours and implementing effective strategies for managing them, you can stay on track with your goals and achieve long-term success. Remember to practice self-compassion, plan ahead, and reach out for support when needed.

Key Points from Step 10: Managing Cravings and Emotional Eating

1. Cravings and emotional eating can negatively impact health by leading to weight gain, poor nutrition, and increased risk of chronic diseases.
2. Mindful eating can help identify triggers for cravings and emotional eating, as well as prevent overeating.
3. Healthy alternatives, such as fruits and vegetables, can be used to manage cravings and improve overall nutrition.
4. Alternative coping mechanisms, such as relaxation techniques or physical activity, can be used to manage emotional eating.
5. Practicing self-compassion and planning ahead can help individuals manage cravings and emotional eating and achieve long-term success in improving their diet and health.

Step 11: Sleep is a Secret Superpower- How Quality Sleep Can Improve your Diet and Health.

Quality sleep is crucial for maintaining good health and making healthy food choices. A lack of sleep quality can make you crave and want to consume high calorie, high fat and high sugar foods. Understanding the importance that good quality sleep can improve your diet choices and health is crucial for long term success:

Reduces Cravings for Unhealthy Foods: Lack of sleep has been linked to increased cravings for unhealthy foods. Some studies have found that individuals who slept for only four hours per night had higher levels of ghrelin, a hormone that stimulates appetite, and lower levels of leptin, a hormone that signals fullness, than those who slept for eight hours per night. This hormonal imbalance can lead to increased cravings for unhealthy foods high in sugar, fat, and calories. Getting adequate sleep can help regulate these hormones, reducing cravings for unhealthy foods and promoting better food choices.

Increases Willpower and Self-Control: Research has shown that sleep deprivation can impair cognitive function, decision-making abilities, and self-control. A study published in the journal Obesity found that sleep-deprived individuals consumed more calories from high-fat and high-sugar foods and had reduced levels of self-control compared to those who slept for the recommended amount of time. Getting adequate sleep can improve cognitive function and decision-making abilities, increasing willpower and self-control, which can help you resist unhealthy food choices and stick to your healthy eating plan.

Promotes Healthy Eating Habits: Quality sleep has been linked to improved mental health, reduced stress, and better mood. A study published in the Journal of Sleep Research found that individuals who slept for less than six hours per night had a higher risk of developing depression and anxiety. Improving mental health and reducing stress can help promote healthy eating habits, such as choosing nutrient-dense foods, preparing healthy meals, and avoiding emotional eating.

Improves Metabolism: Sleep deprivation has been linked to impaired glucose metabolism and insulin resistance, which can increase the risk of obesity and type 2 diabetes. Some studies have found that sleep loss can lead to changes in appetite-regulating hormones, decreased insulin sensitivity, and increased inflammation, all of which can contribute to metabolic dysfunction. Quality sleep helps to regulate metabolism, promoting healthy weight management and reducing the risk of chronic diseases.

Enhances Digestion: Sleep is essential for proper digestion and gut health. There is evidence that sleep deprivation can disrupt the gut microbiome, leading to inflammation, altered nutrient absorption, and impaired digestion. Quality sleep is important for repairing and restoring gut tissue, promoting healthy digestion and nutrient absorption.

Boosts Energy Levels: Adequate sleep is essential for maintaining energy levels throughout the day. Sleep-deprived individuals generally have decreased energy levels and were more likely to consume high-calorie, low-nutrient foods compared to those who slept for the recommended amount of time. Regular physical activity can improve diet choices and overall health, and getting adequate sleep can provide the energy needed to engage in physical activity.

Good sleep hygiene is important for maintaining overall health and well-being. Poor sleep can have negative effects on our physical and mental health, including increasing the risk of chronic conditions such as obesity, diabetes, and heart disease, and contributing to mood disorders like depression and anxiety. In contrast, getting enough quality sleep can help to boost our immune system, improve cognitive function, and enhance our ability to cope with stress.

Improving Sleep To Improve Diet and Heath

The following sleep hygiene tips will help improve the quality and quantity of your sleep which can have a positive effect on your diet choices and overall health:

Stick to a regular sleep schedule: Try to go to bed and wake up at the same time every day, even on weekends. This helps to regulate your body's internal clock and promote better sleep.

Create a relaxing bedtime routine: Develop a relaxing bedtime routine to help signal to your body that it's time to wind down and get ready for sleep. This might include activities such as reading a book, taking a warm bath, or practicing relaxation techniques like deep breathing or meditation.

Sleep Environment: Make sure your sleep environment is conducive to sleep: Ensure that your bedroom is cool, quiet, and dark. Use curtains or blinds to block out any unwanted light and consider using earplugs or a white noise machine to help drown out any background noise.

You nay want to think about investing in a comfortable mattress as well. One study that identified a poor mattress as the top reason for poor sleep in the UK was conducted by the consumer research organization, Which?. In 2017, Which? surveyed over 7,000 UK adults to investigate factors that affect sleep quality. The results of the study were published in the magazine Which? in September 2017, and indicated that a poor mattress was the most commonly reported cause of sleep problems, with 29% of respondents citing this as a reason for their poor sleep.

Avoid stimulants and Alcohol before bedtime: Avoid consuming caffeine, nicotine, or alcohol in the hours leading up to bedtime, as these can interfere with sleep. Both caffeine and nicotine are stimulants and in some cases have a half life of around 12 hours. Meaning even 12 hours after consumption, half of the amount is still present in the body and can have negative effects on sleep. It would be best not consuming caffeine or nicotine after midday to enhance sleep quality.

The use of alcohol traditionally as a 'night cap' to aid sleep unfortunately has terrible consequences and ultimately is back for sleep quality. Alcohol can negatively affect sleep in several ways. Firstly, it can disrupt the natural sleep cycle by reducing the amount of time spent in restorative REM sleep. This can lead to poorer sleep quality, reduced sleep efficiency, and increased daytime sleepiness. Additionally, alcohol can cause breathing problems during sleep, such as snoring or sleep apnoea, which can further disrupt sleep and lead to feelings of fatigue and drowsiness during the day. Alcohol can also affect the body's natural production of hormones such as melatonin, which helps regulate sleep-wake cycles, leading to further disturbances in sleep patterns. Alcohol has been shown to increase the frequency and intensity of night-time wakefulness, leading to a feeling of unrefreshed sleep upon waking. Overall, while alcohol may initially make you feel drowsy and help you fall asleep faster, it can have negative effects on the quality and restorative aspects of sleep.

Limit exposure to screens: The blue light emitted by electronic devices such as smartphones, tablets, and laptops can interfere with sleep by suppressing the production of melatonin. Try to avoid using these devices for at least an hour before bed or consider using a blue light filter or wearing blue light-blocking glasses.

Exercise regularly: Regular physical activity can help to improve the quality of your sleep. Exercise can help regulate the body's natural circadian rhythms, which controls the sleep-wake cycle. Regular exercise can help promote a more consistent sleep schedule, making it easier to fall asleep and wake up at the same time each day. Also, exercise can help reduce stress and anxiety, which are common contributors to sleep problems. However, it's important to avoid exercising too close to bedtime, as this can actually make it harder to fall asleep with the release of certain hormones.

Watch what you eat and drink: Heavy meals and spicy foods can cause indigestion and make it difficult to sleep, so it's best to avoid eating large meals before bedtime. Its recommended eating no later than 2/3 hours before your planned bed time, to give your body time to digest before going to sleep. Similarly, drinking too much fluid before bed can lead to night-time awakenings to use the bathroom.

Quality sleep is essential for maintaining good health and making healthy food choices. By reducing cravings for unhealthy foods, increasing willpower and self-control, promoting healthy eating habits, improving metabolism and digestion, and boosting energy levels, quality sleep can help improve overall health and well-being. There is an abundance of research that supports the important role of sleep in promoting healthy eating habits and reducing the risk of chronic diseases. Aim for at least 7-8 hours of quality sleep per night to optimize your health and support your healthy eating habits.

Key Points from Step 11: Sleep is a Secret Superpower- How Quality Sleep Can Improve Your Diet and Health.

1. Lack of quality sleep can increase cravings for unhealthy foods and lead to hormonal imbalances.
2. Sleep deprivation can impair cognitive function, decision-making abilities, and self-control, reducing willpower and self-control and leading to unhealthy food choices.
3. Quality sleep has been linked to improved mental health, reduced stress, and better mood, promoting healthy eating habits.
4. Sleep deprivation has been linked to impaired glucose metabolism and insulin resistance, which can increase the risk of obesity and type 2 diabetes.
5. Quality sleep is essential for proper digestion and gut health and provides the energy needed to engage in physical activity.

Step 12: Making Nourishment Sustainable: Tips for Long-Term Success

To truly transform your diet and boost your health, it's important to make healthy eating sustainable for the long term. In this chapter, we will explore tips and strategies for making nourishment a sustainable part of your lifestyle.

Understanding the Importance of Sustainability

Many people make the mistake of following short-term diets or fads, which may produce quick results but are difficult to sustain over time. Unfortunately many industries Including the one I work in, the fitness industry can push and sell fad diets to make a quick profit. But if you really want long term meaningful results, it needs to be sustainable. Sustainability means finding a way of eating that works for your lifestyle, preferences, and goals, and that you can maintain over time. Here are a few reasons why sustainability is important:

It's more likely to lead to long-term success: When you find a way of eating that works for you and that you enjoy, you're more likely to stick with it in the long run.

It's healthier: Short-term diets or fads may cut out certain food groups or nutrients, which can lead to deficiencies or imbalances in the long run. A sustainable way of eating should focus on whole, nutrient-dense foods that provide your body with the nutrients it needs to function optimally.

It's more enjoyable: Eating should be a pleasurable experience, and finding a way of eating that you enjoy can make it more sustainable and enjoyable in the long run.

Tips for Making Healthy Eating Sustainable

Here are some tips and strategies for making healthy eating sustainable for the long term:

Focus on Whole, Nutrient-Dense Foods: One of the most important aspects of sustainable healthy eating is focusing on whole, nutrient-dense foods. These foods provide your body with the nutrients it needs to function optimally and support overall health. Some examples of whole, nutrient-dense foods include:

Fruits and vegetables: Aim to eat a variety of fruits and vegetables in a range of colors to ensure you're getting a wide range of nutrients.

Whole grains: Opt for whole grains like brown rice, quinoa, and whole wheat bread instead of refined grains.

Lean protein: Choose lean sources of protein like chicken, fish, tofu, or legumes.

Healthy fats: Include sources of healthy fats like nuts, seeds, avocado, and olive oil in your diet.

Plan and Prep Ahead

Planning and prepping meals and snacks ahead of time can save you time and money, reduce food waste, and help you avoid unhealthy food choices when you're short on time. Here are some tips and strategies for planning and prepping ahead:

Batch cooking: Cook a large batch of a healthy meal, like chili or soup, and portion it out for the week.

Use a slow cooker: Slow cookers are a great way to prepare healthy meals with minimal effort. You can throw in ingredients in the morning and have a hot, healthy meal ready by dinner time.

Prep veggies and fruits in advance: Wash and chop veggies and fruits in advance so they're ready to go when you need them.

Listen to Your Body

Eating in response to physical hunger, rather than emotional or external triggers, is key to making healthy eating sustainable. Here are some tips for practicing mindful eating:

Eat slowly: Take your time when eating and savour each bite.

Pay attention to how you feel: Check in with your hunger and fullness levels before, during, and after eating.

Savour your food: Focus on the flavours, textures, and aromas of your food.

Make Healthy Eating Enjoyable

Eating should be an enjoyable experience, and finding pleasure in healthy eating can make it more sustainable in the long run. Here are some ideas to help you achieve that:

Experiment with new recipes: Trying new recipes and exploring new flavours can make healthy eating more exciting and enjoyable.

Make it social: Eating with friends and family can make healthy eating more enjoyable and create a sense of community around healthy habits. Bring eating around a dining table rather than a TV.

Treat yourself: Including small indulgences in your diet, like a piece of dark chocolate or a glass of wine, can make healthy eating more enjoyable and sustainable in the long run.

Find Support and Accountability

Having support and accountability can be crucial for making healthy eating sustainable in the long run. Here are some ways to find support and accountability:

Enlist a friend or family member to be your accountability partner: Share your goals and progress with someone you trust and who can support and encourage you.

Find Support: Online or in-person support groups or even an accountability coach can provide a sense of community and accountability around healthy eating habits.

Work with a registered dietitian: If you really are struggling or have some serious health issues and intolerances around food, a registered dietitian can provide personalized guidance and support to help you make healthy eating sustainable and maybe needed.

Overcoming Obstacles and Staying Motivated

While adopting a healthy eating pattern can have numerous benefits, it's not always easy to stick to it. Life can throw a variety of challenges your way, such as busy schedules, social events, and cravings, making it difficult to stay on track. Even with the best intentions and strategies, there are common obstacles that can get in the way of making healthy eating sustainable in the long run. Here are some strategies for overcoming these obstacles:

There are things you can do to help you overcome obstacles and stay motivated on your journey to nourishing your body, transforming your diet, and boosting your health.

Plan for Challenges: One of the best ways to overcome obstacles is to plan for them. Think ahead and anticipate any potential challenges that may arise. For example, if you have a busy week ahead, plan your meals and snacks in advance, and prepare some healthy options to grab on the go. If you have a social event coming up, consider eating a healthy snack beforehand, so you're not tempted to indulge in unhealthy foods. If you're eating out look at the menu in advance and plan your choices around the rest of the day.

Practice Self-Compassion: It's essential to practice self-compassion on your journey to better diet. Remember that setbacks and slip-ups are a normal part of the process, and they don't mean you've failed. Instead of beating yourself up over a less-than-perfect meal or snack, be kind to yourself, and focus on getting back on track.

Find Motivation

Staying motivated can be challenging, especially when you've been following a healthy eating pattern for a while. Here are some ways to stay motivated as you go through health and wellbeing journey:

Set realistic goals: Set small, achievable goals for yourself, and celebrate your progress along the way.

Focus on the benefits: Keep reminding yourself of the benefits of healthy eating, such as increased energy, improved mood, and better overall health.

Find inspiration: Look for inspiration in others who have successfully adopted a healthy eating pattern or seek out inspiring recipes or food blogs.

Don't Be Too Hard on Yourself

Remember that no one is perfect, and it's okay to indulge in your favourite foods from time to time. Don't be too hard on yourself for enjoying a treat or for missing a workout. Instead, focus on the bigger picture and how you can continue to make positive food and nutritional choices a sustainable part of your lifestyle.

Get Back on Track

If you do experience a setback, don't give up. Instead, use it as an opportunity to learn and grow. Reflect on what happened and figure out what you can do differently next time. Remember that making nourishment sustainable is a journey, and it's okay to take things one day at a time.

Overcoming obstacles and staying motivated on your journey to transforming your diet and changing your life can be challenging, but it's possible with the right mindset and strategies. By planning for challenges, practicing self-compassion, finding motivation, and getting back on track when things don't go as planned, you can develop a sustainable healthy eating pattern that works for you and your lifestyle.

Making positive and sustainable nutritional choices for the long term is crucial for transforming your diet and boosting your health. By following the tips and strategies outlined in this chapter, you can develop a healthy eating pattern that works for you and your lifestyle. This includes focusing on whole, nutrient-dense foods, planning, and prepping ahead, listening to your body, making healthy eating enjoyable, and finding support.

Remember, developing a sustainable healthy eating pattern is a journey, not a destination. It's okay to make mistakes and have setbacks along the way. The key is to practice self-compassion, get back on track, and keep moving forward. By doing so, you'll be able to nourish your body with the nutrients it needs to feel and function at its best.

Key Points from Step 12: Making Nourishment Sustainable: Tips for Long-Term Success

1. Understanding the importance of sustainability: It's important to find a way of eating that works for your lifestyle, preferences, and goals and that you can maintain over time. It's more likely to lead to long-term success, healthier and more enjoyable.
2. Tips for making healthy eating sustainable: Focus on whole, nutrient-dense foods; plan and prep ahead; listen to your body; make healthy eating enjoyable; find support and accountability.
3. Focus on whole, nutrient-dense foods: Fruits and vegetables, whole grains, lean protein, and healthy fats are essential for sustainable healthy eating.
4. Listen to your body: Eating in response to physical hunger, rather than emotional or external triggers, is key to making healthy eating sustainable.
5. Overcoming obstacles and staying motivated: Planning for challenges, setting achievable goals, and finding alternative healthy options are strategies to overcome obstacles and stay motivated in the journey to a nourishing diet.

Step 13: The Power of Movement: Incorporating Exercise and Movement into Your Life

In today's sedentary world, where many people spend hours sitting in front of a computer or TV, incorporating exercise and movement into your daily routine is more important than ever. Exercise and movement offer numerous physical and mental health benefits, complementing a healthy diet to promote overall health and well-being. In this chapter, we will discuss in detail the importance of exercise and movement, the types of exercises available, and tips for making exercise and movement a regular part of your life.

Benefits of Exercise and Movement

Regular exercise and movement offer numerous benefits for your physical and mental health. Physical benefits include improved cardiovascular health, weight management, reduced risk of chronic diseases, and improved bone density. Exercise and movement also provide mental health benefits, such as reduced stress and anxiety, improved mood, and better cognitive function including improved brain function and memory. In addition, exercise and movement can also help with sleep, reducing the risk of depression, and boosting energy levels.

Types of Exercise and Movement

There are different types of exercises that you can incorporate into your routine, each with its unique benefits. Aerobic exercise, such as running, walking, and cycling, is great for improving cardiovascular health, burning calories, and improving endurance. This type of exercise is ideal for people who want to increase their stamina and endurance, as well as those who want to lose weight.

Strength training, including weightlifting and bodyweight exercises, can help you build muscle mass, increase strength, and improve your metabolism. Strength training exercises are beneficial for people of all ages, but they are particularly important for those over 50, as they can help combat age-related muscle loss and improve bone density.

Flexibility and balance exercises, such as yoga and Pilates, help improve posture, flexibility, and balance. These exercises are beneficial for people of all ages and can help prevent falls in older adults.

Incorporating Exercise and Movement into Your Life

If you're just starting, it's essential to set realistic goals and create a plan that works for you. Finding activities, you enjoy and making movement a part of your daily routine is key to making exercise and movement sustainable. Setting aside time each day for exercise and making it a priority in your schedule can help ensure that you stick to your routine.

When starting an exercise program, it's essential to start slowly and gradually increase the intensity and duration of your workouts. It's also important to incorporate variety into your routine, alternating between different types of exercises to prevent boredom and improve overall fitness.

Overcoming barriers, such as lack of time or motivation, can be challenging, but finding ways to stay motivated, such as setting achievable goals and rewarding yourself when you meet them, can help keep you on track. You can also find support from family, friends, or a personal trainer to help keep you motivated and accountable.

Making Movement Fun and Social

Incorporating exercise and movement into your social life can make it more enjoyable and help keep you motivated. Joining a group fitness class, exercising with a friend or partner, can make exercise and movement more social and fun and ultimately help you stay consistent and accountable.

You can also use technology to make exercise and movement more enjoyable, such as using fitness apps to track your progress.

Staying Safe During Exercise

While exercise and movement offer numerous benefits, it's important to keep safety in mind. It's crucial to start slowly, especially if you're new to exercise, to prevent injury. Proper form and technique are also essential to avoid injury and ensure that you're getting the most out of your workouts.

If you have any medical conditions, it's important to speak with your doctor before starting an exercise program. Your doctor can provide guidance on the types of exercises that are safe for you and any precautions you should take.

It's also important to listen to your body during exercise and stop if you experience any pain or discomfort. Rest and recovery are essential components of any exercise program, and giving your body time to recover can help prevent injury and improve overall performance.

Incorporating exercise and movement into your daily routine is essential for promoting overall health and well-being. The benefits of exercise and movement are numerous, including improved physical and mental health, increased energy levels, and better cognitive function. With the right mindset, planning, and support, anyone can make exercise and movement a regular part of their life and enjoy the many benefits that come with it.

Key Points from Step 13: The Power of Movement: Incorporating Exercise and Movement into Your Life

1. Regular exercise and movement provide numerous physical and mental health benefits, including improved cardiovascular health, weight management, reduced risk of chronic diseases, reduced stress and anxiety, improved mood, and better cognitive function.
2. There are different types of exercises available, including aerobic exercise, strength training, and flexibility and balance exercises, each with its unique benefits.
3. Incorporating exercise and movement into your daily routine requires setting realistic goals, finding activities you enjoy, gradually increasing intensity and duration, incorporating variety, and seeking support from family, friends, or a personal trainer.
4. Making exercise and movement more enjoyable and social can help keep you motivated, such as joining a group fitness class or exercising with a friend or partner.
5. Safety is essential during exercise and movement, requiring starting slowly, using proper form and technique, speaking with a doctor if you have medical conditions, and listening to your body and stopping if you experience any pain or discomfort.

Step 14: Conclusion, Celebrating Your Successes and Continuing to Nourish Your Body

Congratulations on completing this book and taking steps towards transforming your diet and boosting your health! This final chapter will summarize the key takeaways from the book and provide guidance on how to continue nourishing your body, transforming your diet, and boosting your health for the long-term.

Key Takeaways

Throughout this book, we have covered a lot of ground, from understanding the benefits of nourishing your body to strategies for making healthy eating enjoyable, overcoming obstacles, and incorporating exercise into your life. You will have noticed that each chapter whilst focusing on a different area there are lots of reoccurring themes.

- ✓ Set Goals
- ✓ Plan & Prep
- ✓ Make Small Gradual Changes
- ✓ Show Patience and Consistency
- ✓ Eat Nutrient Dense Foods
- ✓ Prioritise Health, Nutrition, Exercise & Sleep

Whilst it may seem like mindless repetition, believe me, it isn't. These themes over arch everything and are crucial for overall success regardless of what.

Continuing to Nourish Your Body

Now that you have a solid understanding of the benefits of nourishing your body and the strategies for achieving a healthy, balanced diet and lifestyle, it's important to continue practicing these habits for long-term success. To continue to nourish your body:

- ✓ Set new goals and challenges for yourself to keep things interesting, engaging and to motivate you to continually improve.
- ✓ Continue to experiment with new foods and recipes to keep your diet diverse and enjoyable.

- ✓ Persevere with goals and remain consistent.
- ✓ Incorporate movement and exercise into your daily routine to improve physical and mental health. Build upon your strength and fitness.
- ✓ Practice mindfulness and stress-management techniques to support overall well-being.
- ✓ Surround yourself with a supportive community that encourages and motivates you to stay on track with your healthy habits.

Transforming your diet and boosting your health is a journey that requires dedication, patience, and support. By implementing the strategies outlined in this book, you can take steps towards achieving optimal health and well-being. Remember to celebrate your successes along the way and continue to nourish your body for the long-term benefit of your health and wellbeing. Best of luck on your journey!

References

Broussard, J. L., Kilkus, J. M., Delebecque, F., Abraham, V., Day, A., Whitmore, H. R., Tasali, E., & Van Cauter, E. (2016). Elevated ghrelin predicts food intake during experimental sleep restriction. Obesity, 24(1), 132–138.

Cosgrove, M. C., Franco, M. N., Natarajan, A. C., Ustunol, T. B., & Capodice, J. B. (2007). Dietary nutrient intake and skin aging appearance among middle-aged American women. Journal of Investigative Dermatology, 127(12), 2880-2889.

David, L. A., Maurice, C. F., Carmody, R. N., Gootenberg, D. B., Button, J. E., Wolfe, B. E., Ling, A. V., Devlin, A. S., Varma, Y., Fischbach, M. A., Biddinger, S. B., Dutton, R. J., & Turnbaugh, P. J. (2014). Diet rapidly and reproducibly alters the human gut microbiome. Nature, 505(7484), 559-563

Donnelly, J. E., Blair, S. N., Jakicic, J. M., Manore, M. M., Rankin, J. W., & Smith, B. K. (2009). American College of Sports Medicine Position Stand. Appropriate physical activity intervention strategies for weight loss and prevention of weight regain for adults. Medicine and Science in Sports and Exercise, 41(2), 459-471.

Ebrahim, I. O., Shapiro, C. M., Williams, A. J., & Fenwick, P. B. (2013). Alcohol and sleep I: Effects on normal sleep. Alcoholism: Clinical and Experimental Research, 37(4), 539-549

Friedenreich, C. M., Cust, A. E., & Lahmann, P. H. (2011). Physical activity and cancer prevention: A review of current evidence. Cancer Causes & Control, 22(6), 811-836.

GBD 2017 Diet Collaborators. (2019). Global, regional, and national comparative risk assessment of 84 behavioural, environmental and occupational, and metabolic risks or clusters of risks for 195 countries and territories, 1990-2017: a systematic analysis for the Global Burden of Disease Study 2017. The Lancet.

Grandner, M. A., Jackson, N. J., Pak, V. M., & Gehrman, P. R. (2012). Sleep disturbance is associated with cardiovascular and metabolic disorders. Journal of Sleep Research, 21(4), 427–433.

Greer, S. M., Goldstein, A. N., & Walker, M. P. (2013). The impact of sleep deprivation on food desire in the human brain. Nature Communications, 4(1), 2259.

Irwin, M. R., & Vitiello, M. V. (2019). Implications of sleep disturbance and inflammation for Alzheimer's disease dementia. The Lancet Neurology, 18(3), 296–306.

Jaiswal, S., & Bauer, H. H. (2019). Vitamin E and skin health. International Journal of Molecular Sciences, 20(22), 5426.

Ley, R. E., Turnbaugh, P. J., Klein, S., & Gordon, J. I. (2006). Microbial ecology: Human gut microbes associated with obesity. Nature, 444(7122), 1022-1023.

Marques-Lopes, I., Ansorena, D., Astiasarán, I., & Forga, L. (2016). Influence of changes in sleep duration on eating behaviour and energy balance. Appetite, 105, 156–164.

Public Health England. (2021). Eatwell Plate. [Image]. Retrieved from https://www.nhs.uk/live-well/eat-well/the-eatwell-guide/

Rao, T. S. S., Asha, M. R., Ramesh, B. N., & Rao, K. S. J. (2008). Understanding nutrition, depression and mental illnesses. Indian Journal of Psychiatry, 50(2), 77–82.

World Health Organization. (2010). Global recommendations on physical activity for health. https://www.who.int/publications/i/item/9789241599979